Type 1 Diabetes

All you need to know

Dr. Sheila Harrison

Disclaimer

This content is not a substitute for consulting a professional physician but to give a fair knowledge about the disease and to equip you to seek medical assistance as early as possible if need be to avoid complications. It should also be noted that the area of medical science is a constantly changing field and due to the ever developing and changing nature of medical knowledge, we suggest you seek expert advice if you spot any discrepancies or decide to take action in reaction to the information in this content. Never reject medical advice from professionals or put off getting treatment because of something you read online, acquired through this material, or any other online resource.

And remember the internet won't heal you but God through Physicians will.

Table of contents

Introduction

Type 1 diabetes is a chronic autoimmune disorder that affects the lives of millions of individuals worldwide. It arises from the intricate interplay between genetic and environmental factors. This leads to the destruction of insulin-producing beta cells within the area in the pancreas called pancreatic islets of Langerhans. Unlike type 2 diabetes, type 1 diabetes is an autoimmune response that targets the body's own insulin - producing cells.

Previously known as juvenile diabetes due to its onset mostly in childhood and adolescence, type 1 diabetes can occur at any age. But it usually starts in kids and teens. However, now, we're seeing more adults getting type 1 diabetes too. It places a substantial physical, emotional, and economic burden on individuals, families, and healthcare systems. The dependence on insulin, the risk of hypoglycemia and hyperglycemia, and the potential long-term complications increase the need for more research to understand the disease and its effective treatment strategies better.

Type 1 diabetes can affect people from different places and backgrounds. Also, the number of people with type 1 diabetes varies in different countries and groups of people. The World Health Organization (WHO) suggests that the number of type 1 diabetes is increasing globally in recent years.

This article aims to provide a comprehensive overview of the complex mechanisms of type 1 diabetes, studying its symptoms, causes, diagnosis, and treatment, and reviewing the latest research. This knowledge, in the end, can enhance the quality of life for those dealing with this demanding condition.

Section 1

What are the causes of type 1 diabetes?

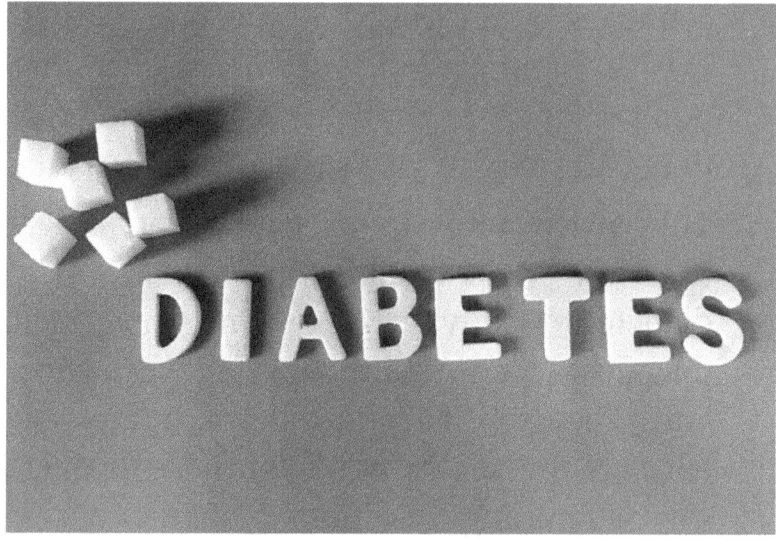

Understanding the causes of type 1 diabetes is a complex challenge. It involves understanding the intricate interplay of genetics and environmental triggers. This section delves into the multifaceted factors contributing to the development of this autoimmune condition.

Genetic factors

Human leukocyte antigen (HLA) region:
A big part of why some people are more likely to get type 1 diabetes is because of certain genes that are in charge of the body's defense system. These genes are like the commanders of the army that protects our bodies. Sometimes, changes in these genes can make a person more likely to have diabetes.

There are special types of these genes, such as HLA-DR3 and HLA-DR4. Researchers found these genes to make it easier for diabetes to happen. These genes affect how our defense system works. They can also make it go after the cells that make insulin. We need to control our blood sugar.

Non-HLA Genes (INS, PTPN22, CTLA4, etc.):
While HLA genes are key players, the genetic landscape of type 1 diabetes extends beyond the HLA region. Numerous non-HLA genes also contribute to the risk of developing the disease. These genes include insulin (INS), protein tyrosine phosphatase non-receptor type 22

(PTPN22), cytotoxic T-lymphocyte-associated protein 4 (CTLA4), and others. Variations in these genes affect immune function, insulin regulation, and other crucial pathways involved in maintaining self-tolerance.

Environmental triggers

Viral infections

Environmental factors play a vital role in triggering the onset of Type 1 diabetes in genetically predisposed people. Researchers have suspected viral infections among these environmental factors as potential triggers for a long time. Certain viruses, such as enteroviruses and coxsackieviruses, have been implicated in initiating the autoimmune response against beta cells. These viruses may start an abnormal immune reaction, leading to the destruction of insulin-producing cells. The mechanisms by which viral infections contribute to the development of type 1 diabetes are complex. And it also involves interactions between viral components and the immune system.

Early childhood nutrition

The impact of early childhood nutrition on type 1 diabetes development is an emerging area of research. Evidence suggests that factors such as breastfeeding duration, introduction of solid foods, and composition of an infant's diet may influence the risk of the disease. Nutritional components, such as vitamin D and omega-3 fatty acids, have been studied for their potential protective effects against type 1 diabetes. Exploring these nutritional influences provides insight into modifiable factors that could mitigate disease risk.

Gut microbiota

Gut microbiota is a complex ecosystem of microorganisms residing in the gastrointestinal tract. It has garnered attention for its potential role in autoimmune diseases including type 1 diabetes. Emerging research suggests that alterations in gut microbiota composition and diversity may impact immune function as well as contribute to the breakdown of immune tolerance. Dysbiosis in the gut microbiome could potentially trigger immune responses that target beta cells. Investigating the intricate relationship between gut microbiota and type 1 diabetes offers new avenues for understanding disease development and potential therapeutic interventions.

Section 2

What are the symptoms of type 1 diabetes?

Type 1 diabetes shows a distinct set of symptoms that arise from the abnormal production of insulin. Individuals may experience polyuria or excessive urination because the kidneys work to eliminate excess glucose from the bloodstream. This leads to polydipsia or intense thirst because the body attempts to counteract fluid loss. Weight loss, despite increased appetite, can occur due to the breakdown of fats and proteins for energy in the absence of sufficient glucose utilization. Fatigue and weakness may result from the body's inability to properly utilize nutrients. Blurred vision, caused by changes in fluid balance within the eye's lens, is another hallmark symptom. As the disease progresses, untreated type 1 diabetes can lead to a life-threatening condition known as diabetic ketoacidosis (DKA). It is characterized by elevated blood ketone levels, metabolic acidosis, as well as potential organ dysfunction.

Section 3

How is type 1 diabetes diagnosed?

The diagnosis of type 1 diabetes relies on clinical symptoms and available laboratory-confirmed tests. According to the American Diabetes Association (ADA), the diagnostic criteria include:

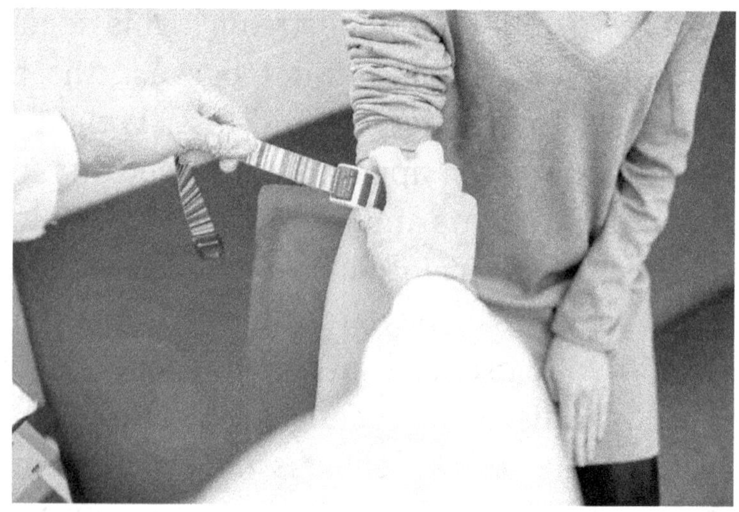

- **Symptoms:** The presence of classic symptoms such as polyuria, polydipsia, and unexplained weight loss.

- **Hyperglycemia:** A random plasma glucose level greater than or equal to 200 mg/dL (11.1 mmol/L), measured in individuals with classic symptoms.

- **Fasting Plasma Glucose:** A fasting plasma glucose level greater than or equal to 126 mg/dL (7.0 mmol/L) after an overnight fast of at least 8 hours.

- **Oral Glucose Tolerance Test (OGTT):** A 2-hour plasma glucose level greater than or equal to 200 mg/dL (11.1 mmol/L) during a 75g oral glucose tolerance test.

- **Autoantibody Markers (ICA, GADA, IA-2A, etc.):** Autoantibody markers serve as valuable tools in confirming the autoimmune nature of Type 1 diabetes and predicting disease progression. Islet cell antibodies (ICA), glutamic acid decarboxylase antibodies (GADA), insulinoma-associated-2 antibodies (IA-2A), and zinc transporter 8 antibodies (ZnT8A) are among the autoantibodies commonly assessed. These antibodies reflect the immune system's attack on beta cells and contribute to the identification of individuals at risk for or in the early stages of type 1 diabetes.

Autoantibody testing provides insight into the likelihood of future beta cell decline, helping doctors in determining appropriate management strategies and monitoring. Positive autoantibody status, coupled with clinical symptoms, may prompt early intervention to optimize glucose control and potentially delay disease progression.

Section 4

How is type 1 diabetes treated?

Managing type 1 diabetes requires a multifaceted approach that aims to mimic physiological insulin secretion, maintain optimal glucose levels, and enhance overall quality of life. Taking care of type 1 diabetes needs a multifaceted approach. The goal is to copy how the body naturally uses insulin, keep your sugar levels just right, and improve your quality of life. This section delves into giving insulin to the body externally, using new tools for insulin, using clever ways to give insulin, and always keeping an eye on your sugar levels. We also look at how the food you eat and how you live your life can help keep your sugar levels in a good range.

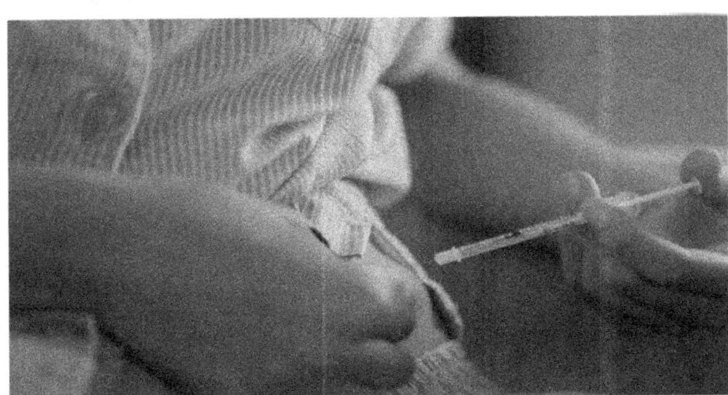

Insulin administration from outside

A cornerstone of type 1 diabetes management involves the replacement of insulin through exogenous administration. There may be some possible side effects of taking insulin during diabetes. However, since the pancreas no longer produces insulin, individuals with type 1 diabetes rely on injected or infused insulin to regulate glucose levels and prevent hyperglycemia. In such a situation, avoiding insulin may not be an option if you have type 1 diabetes.

Insulin types and regimens

A variety of insulin formulations are available, each with distinct characteristics suited to different patient needs. Rapid-acting insulins, such as lispro and aspart, are used to cover meals and correct elevated glucose levels. Long-acting insulins, such as glargine and detemir, provide basal insulin coverage. They mimic the steady background secretion of insulin between meals and during sleep.

Insulin analogues

Insulin analogues have revolutionized diabetes care by copying natural insulin secretion patterns more closely than traditional insulins. These analogues offer rapid start and more predictable durations of action, allowing for greater flexibility in dosing and meal timing.

Insulin delivery systems

Innovations in insulin delivery systems have transformed the way individuals manage their diabetes, enhancing convenience and precision.

Insulin pumps

Insulin pumps are wearable devices that deliver continuous basal insulin through a subcutaneous catheter. They offer customisable insulin dosing. This enables the users to adjust basal rates for different times of day and bolus insulin for meals and corrections.

Insulin pens

Insulin pens provide an alternative to traditional syringes, offering convenient insulin administration. These devices come in both disposable and reusable forms and allow for accurate dosing.

Continuous Glucose Monitoring (CGM)

CGM systems have revolutionized diabetes management by providing real-time data on glucose levels. These devices continuously monitor interstitial glucose levels and transmit the data to a receiver or smartphone. CGM provides insights into glucose trends, which helps users make informed decisions about insulin dosing, exercise, and dietary choices.

Benefits and applications

The benefits of CGM extend beyond glucose monitoring. These systems offer alerts for high and low glucose levels, reducing the risk of severe hypoglycemia and hyperglycemia. CGM data can identify patterns as well as make informed adjustments to insulin regimens and lifestyle choices.

Real-time glucose monitoring

Real-time glucose monitoring empowers individuals with type 1 diabetes so that they are able to make immediate and proactive decisions based on their glucose readings. By continuously tracking glucose levels, users can adjust insulin doses, time meals, and make lifestyle modifications to maintain optimal glycemic control.

Dietary and lifestyle management

Dietary and lifestyle management play important roles in optimizing glucose control and promoting overall well-being for individuals with type 1 diabetes. Carbohydrate counting, portion control, and balanced nutrition are essential components of effective diabetes management. Regular physical activity contributes to improved insulin sensitivity and cardiovascular health.

Psychosocial aspects and quality of life

The management of type 1 diabetes extends beyond the physiological aspects of blood glucose control and insulin administration. A holistic approach also recognizes the psychosocial aspects of living with a chronic condition. The emotional and psychological toll of type 1 diabetes is huge. The daily demands of monitoring blood glucose levels, calculating insulin doses, and navigating the uncertainties of managing the condition can lead to diabetes distress, anxiety, and depression.

So, coping strategies become essential tools for individuals as they navigate the challenges of type 1 diabetes. Problem-focused strategies involve learning practical skills for managing diabetes-related tasks and situations. These strategies include carbohydrate counting, effective insulin dosing, limiting alcohol consumption as well as tobacco, and regular exercise. Emotion-focused strategies address the emotional responses to diabetes, emphasizing mindfulness, stress reduction, and seeking social support. Adaptive coping mechanisms empower individuals to maintain a sense of control and resilience in the face of the condition's demands.

Mental health support

Recognising and addressing the psychological well-being of individuals with type 1 diabetes is essential. Mental health support encompasses a range of interventions aimed at promoting emotional well-being, reducing distress, and enhancing overall quality of life.

Psychological counseling and therapy provide safe spaces for individuals to explore their feelings, develop coping skills, and address diabetes-related challenges. Cognitive-behavioral therapy (CBT) and acceptance and commitment therapy (ACT) are common approaches that empower individuals to reframe negative thought patterns, manage stress, and navigate emotional hurdles.

Peer support groups as well as online communities offer a platform for individuals to connect with others having similar experiences. These forums provide opportunities to share insights, exchange practical tips, and foster a sense of belonging, reducing feelings of isolation.

Integrating mental health support into routine diabetes care ensures that emotional well-being is prioritized alongside physical health. Healthcare providers play a crucial role in assessing psychological needs, providing appropriate referrals, and engaging in open conversations about the psychosocial challenges associated with Type 1 diabetes.

Section 5

What is the future treatment of type 1 diabetes?

The landscape of type 1 diabetes research is evolving, opening up a new era of targeted and innovative therapeutic strategies aimed at reshaping the immune response, preserving beta cell function, and ultimately improving the lives of individuals with the condition. This section delves into immunotherapies and explores potential future directions in type 1 diabetes treatment and prevention.

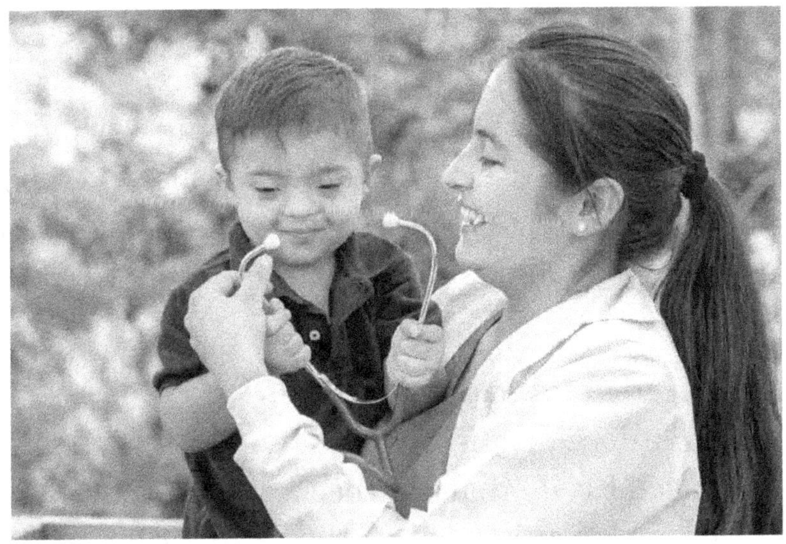

Immune modulation strategies

Immunotherapy approaches for type 1 diabetes seek to restore the normal functions of the immune system, stop the immune system from attacking its own beta cells, and preserve insulin production. Various agents which can affect the functions of the immune system are under investigation to selectively target immune cells and change their activity for good.

A special treatment to stop diabetes

There is a special treatment called antigen-specific immunotherapy. It tries to make the immune system less sensitive to the things that attack beta cells. They give specific parts of these attacking things to the body to help it get used to them. They also use special cells that have been changed to show these attacking things to the immune system.

Stem cells to fix diabetes

Another idea is to use stem cells. These are special cells that can become different types of cells. Scientists think they can turn stem cells into cells that make insulin. These new cells could then be put into the body to replace the ones that were destroyed. They're also trying to find ways to make these new cells survive better and not get attacked by the immune system.

Helper cells to calm the immune system

There are some cells called regulatory T cells that help calm down the immune system and stop it from attacking. Scientists are looking into ways to make more of these cells and make them stronger. They want to use these cells to tell the immune system to stop hurting the beta cells.

Changing genes to fight diabetes

We now have a tool called CRISPR/Cas9 that can change genes. Scientists want to use it to help people with diabetes. They may change the genes in immune cells or in beta cells to protect them better. This could change how we treat diabetes in a big way.

Stopping diabetes before it starts

Instead of just treating diabetes, scientists want to stop it from happening. They're looking at people's genes and special things in the blood to find out who might get diabetes. They're also trying out treatments that could help save the beta cells when they start getting hurt. This is important to catch diabetes early or even prevent it.

Closed-loop systems

Ongoing studies refine closed-loop systems that automate insulin delivery based on real-time glucose monitoring, enhancing glycemic control and reducing the risk of hypoglycemia.

Artificial intelligence

AI-driven algorithms are being integrated into diabetes management platforms to analyze data, predict glucose trends, and optimize insulin dosing.

Implantable insulin delivery devices

Implantable devices, such as microchips or capsules, hold the potential to provide sustained insulin delivery without the need for frequent injections. These devices release insulin in response to glucose levels, mimicking the natural behavior of healthy beta cells.

Inhaled insulin

Inhalable insulin offers an alternative to injections, enabling individuals to deliver insulin via inhalation. This technology provides rapid insulin absorption through the lungs, making it particularly useful for mealtime insulin dosing.

Nanotechnology

Nanoscale technologies are being explored for their potential to improve insulin stability, enhance drug delivery, and reduce injection frequency. Nanoparticles and nanocarriers may facilitate targeted insulin delivery and improve insulin formulations.

Section 6

FAQ on Type 1 Diabetes

Can type 1 diabetes affect kidney diseases?

Type 1 diabetes can lead to diabetic kidney disease (diabetic nephropathy) due to high blood sugar damaging kidney blood vessels and filters. This can cause protein leakage, high blood pressure, inflammation, and nerve damage, potentially leading to kidney dysfunction. Tight blood sugar control, blood pressure management, and regular monitoring are key to preventing or slowing kidney complications.

Can type 1 diabetes affect liver diseases?

Type 1 diabetes can have a limited impact on liver health. It's associated with a slightly higher risk of non-alcoholic fatty liver disease (NAFLD) and autoimmune liver diseases, but this is not as significant as other complications like kidney or heart issues. Maintaining a healthy lifestyle and monitoring blood sugar

27

levels are still important to reduce potential liver-related risks.

Can type 1 diabetes cause heart problems?

Type 1 diabetes can increase the risk of heart problems due to high blood sugar damaging blood vessels, causing atherosclerosis, inflammation, high blood pressure, abnormal lipid levels, nerve damage affecting heart control, and potential heart muscle dysfunction. Managing blood sugar, blood pressure, cholesterol, and a healthy lifestyle are crucial to reduce this risk.

Does high cholesterol cause type 1 diabetes?

No, high cholesterol does not cause type 1 diabetes. Type 1 diabetes is an autoimmune condition where the immune system mistakenly attacks and destroys the insulin-producing cells in the pancreas. High cholesterol, on the other hand, is related to imbalances in lipid levels in the blood and is not a direct cause of type 1 diabetes. However, both high cholesterol and type 1 diabetes can increase the risk of heart problems when they coexist.

Why is type 1 diabetes a sign of weak bones?

Type 1 diabetes can lead to weaker bones due to factors like reduced bone density, hormonal imbalances, chronic inflammation, vitamin D deficiency, certain medications, poor blood sugar control, and reduced physical activity. Maintaining blood sugar control, ensuring proper nutrition, staying physically active, and discussing concerns with a healthcare provider can help mitigate this risk.